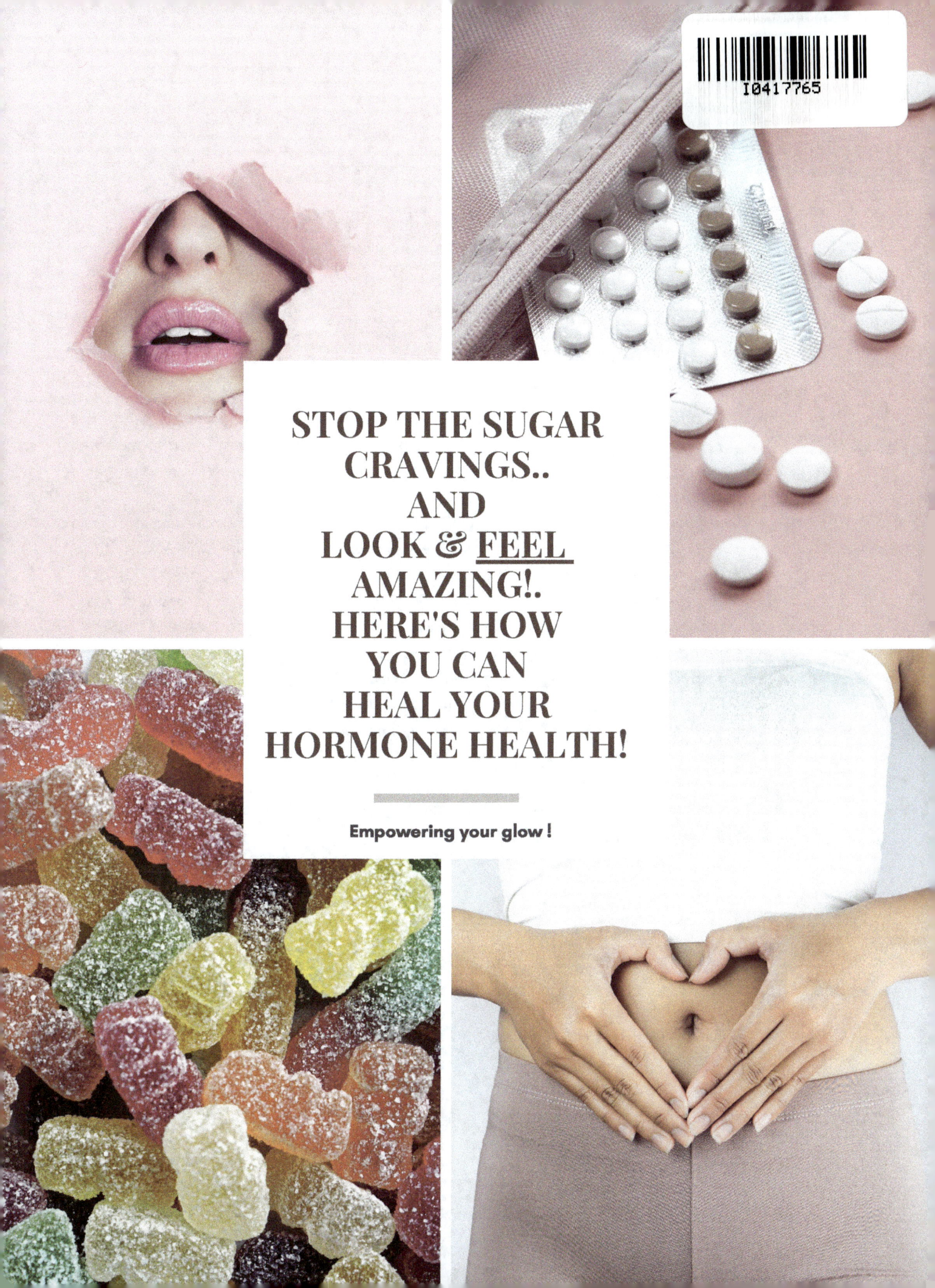

STOP THE SUGAR
CRAVINGS..
AND
LOOK & <u>FEEL</u>
AMAZING!.
HERE'S HOW
YOU CAN
HEAL YOUR
HORMONE HEALTH!

Empowering your glow !

Copyright & Disclaimer

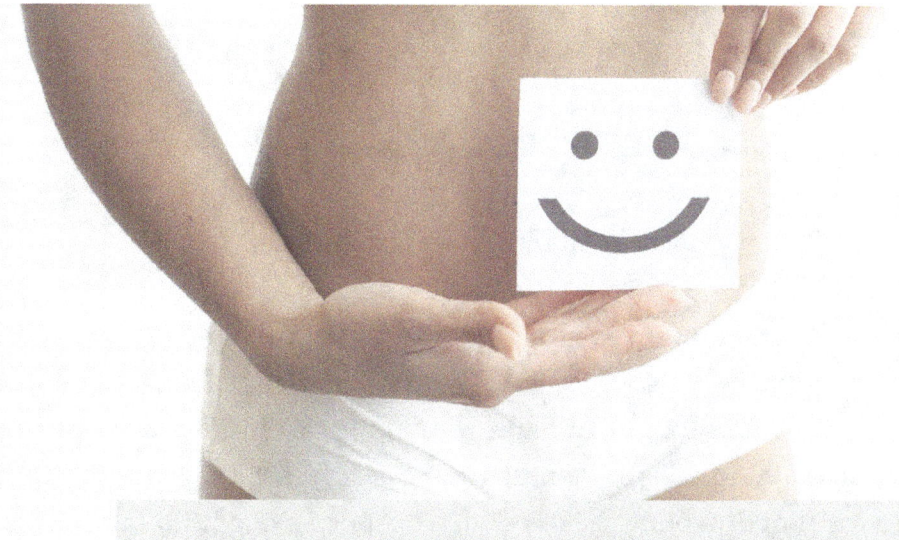

TABLE OF CONTENTS

What is really behind the Sugar Cravings?

Did you know studies have shown that;

Sugar acts in the Brain the same way as Cocaine does! by stimulating the release of Dopamine Neuro transmitters in the same kind of 'High' of Addictive Pleasure as Cocaine. So when people call themselves 'Sugar Addicts' without realising there is a truth in that! Since Sugar has such a strong pull on Mental and Physical Desire it is no wonder it feels almost impossible to resist our favourite Sticky Bun, Cookie or Chocolate Bar and feel like we are defeated by our Sugar Cravings.

We have all likely heard the news that **Sugar can cause Inflammation in our bodies which is directly linked to Serious Illnesses like Cancer, Diabetes and Heart Disease**. To name but a few.

Unfortunately most Processed Food Product Producers are still putting Profits before People since it pays off for them, for us to be addicted to Sugar since we will naturally buy more goods.

Even though **studies have shown than cutting just 20% of Sugar from processed foods could prevent 500,000 deaths.** We need to look after ourselves.

But is it really realistic and viable to go completely Sugar Free?

Diets don't work: 95% of people who have lost Weight Dieting will regain the weight. If you think that most of the foods we eat on a daily basis contain refined Sugar is it any wonder.

We will go through what has been proven to actually work better for longer term Healthy Eating that **Weight Loss and ongoing Weight Maintenance is a Natural Side effect** of. Alongside better **Balanced Hormones** for long term treatment of getting to grips of the root cause behind the Sugar Cravings in this Guide.

But the big Secret that most people do not know, is it can also be our undiagnosed Hormone Imbalances and Gut Health that could be causing the Sugar Cravings. That's how this Guide is Unique and we look at improving your whole Holistic Hormone Health. You will Look and Feel your very Best once this is in Balance.

What is a Hormone Imbalance?

It is more common than you may realise:

47% of Women
are living with
the symptoms of
a Hormone Imbalance

You can blame the Sugar Cravings on your Hormones!. Studies have found that changes in levels of Estrogen and Progesterone are often responsible for causing cravings for high Carb and Sweet Foods. Alongside deficiencies in certain Nutrients if you are regularly craving Sweets & Treats.

Nowadays it is just as frequent to have a Hormone Imbalance than not to be having one, at some time in our lives most often during our 30's and 40's.
Before going into Menopause. Its quite often misunderstood, but to break it down it is generally our Bodies trying to draw our attention to something we need to look at and address with our Health. Surprisingly most often by Natural methods : Diet, Lifestyle or a Detox Plan can set us on the path to recovery and feeling great again in good Health once we have found the cause.

However most people aren't aware of this and can spend years and even decades suffering. Living with an imbalance and can be misdiagnosed or masking it with medication and never addressing the root cause. Of course each case is different and that's why I advocate getting Blood tests done. I have included 'The Secrets to Curbing Cravings' so even if you don't have a Hormone Imbalance and simply need your 'Gut Health' and 'Food Psychology' Detoxing and Resetting it's coming up later!.
The reason I have created this Guide is to use as a starting point to inform and Empower you that life can be great again and even better on the other side!.

Do you have any of these Symptoms?

What is your Body trying to telling you!

Symptoms;

- **Painful Periods**
- **Fatigue**
- **Hair Thinning or Loss**
- **Heightened Emotions**
- **Mood swings**
- **Sugar cravings**
- **Adult Acne and Skin Breakouts**
- **Infertility**
- **Bloating**
- **Gut Health and IBS issues**
- **Weight Gain**
- **Imbalanced Blood Sugars**
- **Low Libido**
- **Hirsutism**
- **Anxiety or Depression**
- **Aggressive or out of the norm Behaviour**

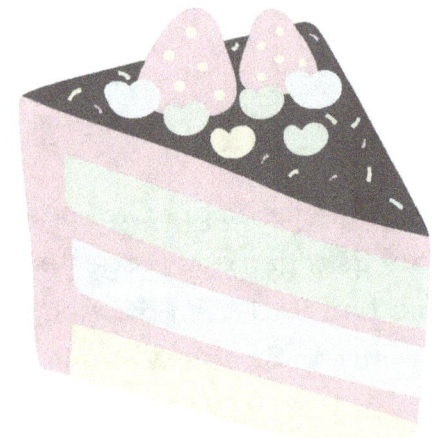

To name but a few of the symptoms of A Hormonal Imbalance. **Even one of these areas could be your Body dealing with an imbalance. This guide will help you to discover and treat 'Hormone Imbalance' naturally. Science has proven Nutrition, Lifestyle and Detox over Medication For dramatically improving or healing most imbalances, once we know what we are dealing with!**

What your 'Period Palette' could be telling you about your Hormone Balance

BRIGHT RED= Normal Healthy Period!. Flow should start moderate (not spotting) and flow like a river and taper off. Low Pain and no PMS

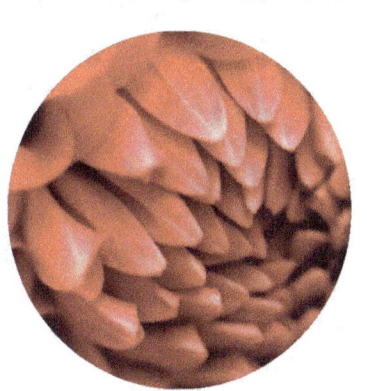

Light Pink= Light Bleeding may indicate Low Estrogen Levels, Extreme Dieting or Exercise or Nutrient Deficiency

Dark Red/Purple

Dark Red with a Purple shade and Heavy Bleeding. Usually with Clots, **PMS + Painfull** can be an indicator of PCOS, Endometriosis, Ovarian Cysts and **Imbalance**

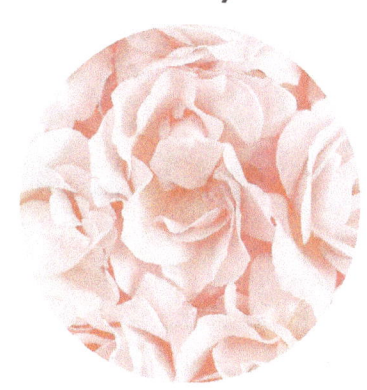

Brownish/ Maroon

Colour may indicate **Low Progesterone ,** can also be old blood from previous cycle.

Orange

Not always but may indicate a sign of Vaginal infection

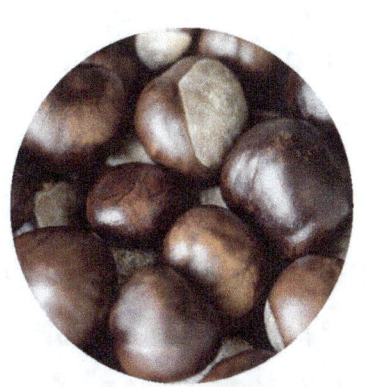

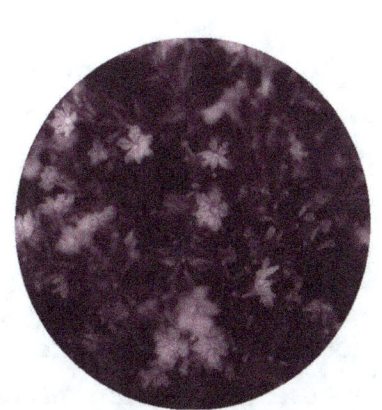

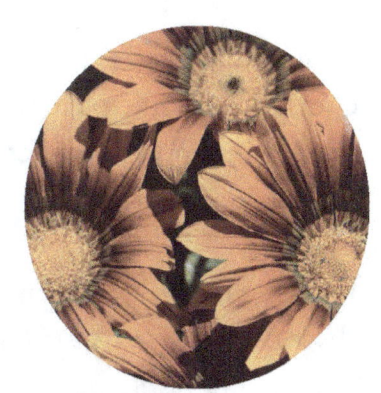

Modern Life Hormone Malfunction

What it is and how it could be impacting your Health in ways you may not even realise!

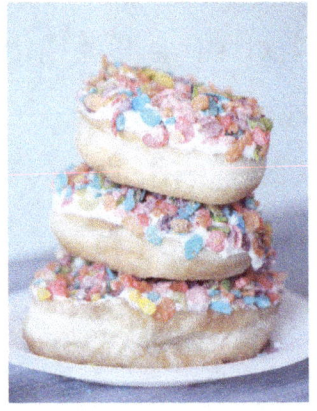 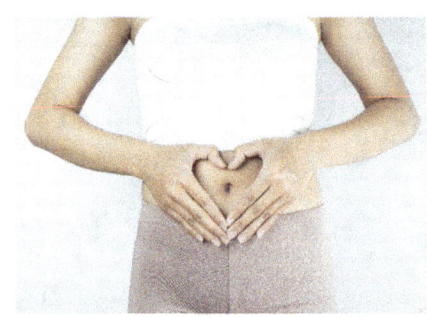 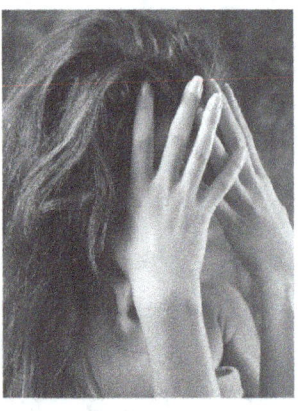

In the past many of the symptoms, caused by Hormones that are out of Balance have often been **overlooked as 'normal' and called names like: 'Women's Issues'**.

These so called 'normal' symptoms are in fact, not normal and you shouldn't have to put up with them!. **They are often a way for our bodies to communicate with us, an early warning sign something is not right. Not only do you not have to put up with them. Some of the symptoms, if left untreated or ignored can even develop into more serious Health issues.**

What's worse is that some of these symptoms are often underestimated, and belittled in the Media and Workplace ; Women feel shamed if they need to miss work or are having a tough day. Or feel they have to battle on regardless.

Fortunately word is getting out about this and the Holistic, Diet and Lifestyle tweaks and changes you can make that have been proven to work as treatments, can be transformational for Mood, Weight, Fertility, Skin, Hair and your Life!. Which we will cover more in this Guide.

Life can be so much better!
Also Menopause doesn't need to be a Nightmare either if this is you? I have a Free guide coming out dedicated to Menopause. Email for details kerry.healthplan@gmail.com

Introduction

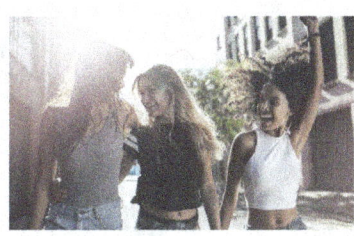

Hello!..

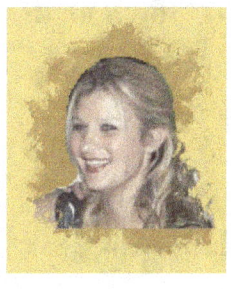

Kerry Goodliffe
Author and
Hormone Health
& Wellness Coach

Are you ready to learn the truth about getting to the Happiest Healthiest, Hottest and Sexiest version of you! Without compromising Health for Beauty!.

I'm so excited, you are potentially about to embark on living your Best & Healthy Life!. I remember 5 years ago **I was suffering with Acne, thinning Hair and couldn't loose Weight but I also had constant Sugar cravings, IBS, Anxiety, Infertility and sadly experienced several Miscarriages**. And like most Women I talk to, I had no idea what was behind it all. **I thought it was normal.** I even experienced a rare type of **Cancer** that took me to undertake a deep dive Research mission into the **Science Journals** because I wasn't been given the answers. I finally got my **Poly Cystic Ovary Syndrome** diagnosis but that was it. There was nobody to help me with this Life altering Metabolic Condition.

In order to help myself I retrained as a **Hormone Health Coach in Nutrition.** Because **what I found and put into place not only helped me get my Insulin Resistance under control and reduce Chemo side effects I was also able to conceive my Miracle Rainbow Babies.** I'm on a Mission to help other Women like you that are at the stage of finding answers and looking for help and answers to piece together what is happening to their Health and that **want to learn how to get control over the symptoms that I myself had also felt I had to put up with before finding how to heal myself!.**

What I have learned about Sugar, Endocrine disruptors and inflammation during my own Cancer diagnosis & Studies was Life Changing. All of these factors meant I wasn't Ovulating regularly enough. And the Science is if that is a regular enough occurrence then:

un-apposed Estrogen can cause an imbalance which is proven to be more likely to increase the risk of a number of Health Issues and even Endometrial Cancers such as mine was. I want to prevent that for as many Women as possible. Sharing what I know and my own Hormone Health & Protection Lifetime Plan in this Guide.

And for those that are trying for a Baby and perhaps experienced Infertility and Miscarriage *see the TTC chapter.* I understand that this can lead us to think we are broken! You are not at Fault! Follow my: **Optimise Natural Fertility Pre Conception Plan** to increase your odds of getting Pregnant faster!

Our Skin & Hormones

How your Skin is affected by your Hormone Balance:

Acne

At any age!

Most acne is caused by excess oil production which clogs the pores in your skin. The Hormone Androgen (in excess) affects many Women, some of the symptoms are Blemishes, PCOS, Sugar Cravings, Anxiety, Mood, Hair issues..

Sebaceous glands on the Skin are very sensitive to Androgens. The more Androgens in your blood, the more oil is produced. Out of balance Oestrogen is also thought to affect the amount of sebum you produce. **Which is why a topical skin care product won't necessarily make a difference.**

Dry Skin Itchy or Irritable skin

Some of the culprits!:

Thyroid hormone

When your thyroid hormone is low, it can cause a number of signs such as dry skin.

Cortisol

Is elevated in times of stress. When your body is in a state of stress, it triggers a response to the inflammatory system, which can cause itching. This is why those with eczema notice "flare-ups" in situations of stress or without realisation of a hormone imbalance.

The last of the hormones related to dry skin is your Progesterone and Estrogen level ratio imbalance can lead to dryness. And is also why during Menopause the effects can be increased as the drop of these Hormones accelerate

What can cause Hormone Imbalance that affects the Skin:

- **Stress**
- **High GI Foods** *(Carbs & Sugars)*
- **Inflammation caused by the above**
- **Poor Sleep** *which will continue until the Hormone Imbalance is addressed.*
- *A Nutrient Deficiency*

Addressing the Natural Balance <u>from within</u> with is more effective than an external Cream or Lotion.

Hair and Hormones

Dry Brittle or Thinning Hair or Itchy Scalp?

Tired of your Products not doing what they claim to do? Save time and Money by Treating the Root Cause..

There are Hormone related factors that can impact the Hair and its growth and condition. These are:

- **Androgen levels**
- **Insulin**
- **Triiodothyronine / Thyroxin- (Thyroid Health)**

All of these can result in dryer hair, thinning hair, Aleopecea and hair loss when the levels are not correctly balanced or kept in check.
The Good news is once we know which area is imbalanced the treatment to improve the underlying problem can start.

**Ready to take the Hormone Health Quiz :
Hormonehealthbliss.com**

Weight and Hormones

The Big Fat Lies of the Weight loss and Diet industry and what really makes a difference to our Weight.

FACT 1

Did you know that high impact & over exercise can actually make Weight Loss harder?

FACT 2

Low fat diets can end up making us fat?

FACT 3

What actually makes a difference to our Weight and how we utilise and store Fat is our Hormone Balance

Hormones Regulate our appetite and signal to our Brains when to eat and when to stop eating.
If something is going on with our Hormones it's also impacting our Metabolism, which is how it starts affecting our Weight and can cause Weight gain.

When we eat processed Foods and added Sugar it can increase levels of Hunger Hormones and numb the effect of fullness Hormone Sensors. These effects may prompt overeating and Weight gain.

Processed foods increases our exposure to endocrine-disrupting chemicals
These chemicals have been shown to alter the hormones that regulate appetite, fullness, and food preferences making us crave even more Sugary, Salty and Fatty foods. And can also cause insulin resistance — all of these factors can influence weight gain.

The place to start is by regulating our cells response to these Hormones and support our natural Metabolism. In many Women, Inositol deficiency has been found to be behind Sugar Cravings and Insulin Resistance. It has been found that many Women actually have a defect in how their body utilises the Inositol they should be getting from foods, which are required for adequate Blood Sugar balance. If this happens on a regular enough basis Insulin Resistance and type 2 Diabetes can develop. By supplementing with supplements that support and rectify the Deficiency such as My Myo Plan's Myo Inositol, research has shown to help the Sugar cravings , restore Hormone balance and reduce the risk of Insulin Resistance in these women.

Ready to take the Hormone Health Quiz? https://hormonehealthbliss.com/hormone-health-quiz

Hormones and our Mood

Our Hormones impact our physical and emotional well-being.
If one type of Hormone is out of balance it has a knock on affect on the rest. Estrogen Dominance and Cortisol imbalance is very common.

The general affects of an Imbalance can cause:
- **Anxiety**
- **Negative thoughts**
- **Prone to Worry more**
- **Difficulty concentrating**
- **Feelings of Guilt**
- **Emotional or Weepy**
- **Angry**
- **Mood Swings**
- **Low Mood or Depression**

These are just a few examples.

How an Imbalance happens:
- **Endocrine Disrupting Chemicals in our Foods or Products (Shampoo, Perfume, Household Cleaning Products)**
- **Stress**
- **Poor Sleep**
- **Sugar, Fat and Salts (Processed Foods)**
- **If the Thyroid is disrupted you become more prone to depression**

Too much Cortisol from Stress can have a negative impact on our immune system, as well as causing weight gain and sleep issues. This in turn can have a negative impact on our moods.

If you are struggling with poor overall Mood, persistent Depression, Anxiety or Mood swings, its going to be beneficial to get your Hormone levels checked. Which you can request from your Doctor or Online. Certain Nutritional deficiencies can cause Mood issues we will go into how to find and address these later in the Guide.

The missing piece of the Puzzle that affects our Hair, Skin, Health & Sleep:
Hormone Imbalance

It is widely accepted that most short term Hormone Imbalances happen just after giving birth or are due to coming off the Birth Control Pill which is often prescribed to mask symptoms but has been proven to often make matters worse later down the line.

The other type of 'long term' Hormone Imbalances can go on far longer disguised in areas in our lives that could be silently there in the background but are sabotaging our Fertility or Weight by our best efforts to stay away from the Biscuit tin or making us break out in Adult Acne. We accept and cover up with cosmetics and potions.
Here are the following triggers:
Stress, An unbalanced Diet, high Sugar intake, Junk food, poor Sleep , Caffeine and Alcohol intake, and a Sedentary Lifestyle.
And what's worse all of these issues can lead our bodies to become more addicted to Sugar that feeds the Inflammation and makes matters worse.

However it has also been found that due to our Modern Lifestyles the average Women now comes into contact with over 200 **Endocrine Disrupting Chemicals** daily. Mainly found in her Make Up, Fragrance and Beauty Products but also around the house, in innocent household products like Soap, Detergent, Cleaning Products and even the Food we eat and the packaging its wrapped in.
Endocrine Disrupting Chemicals.

What are Endocrine Disrupting Chemicals?

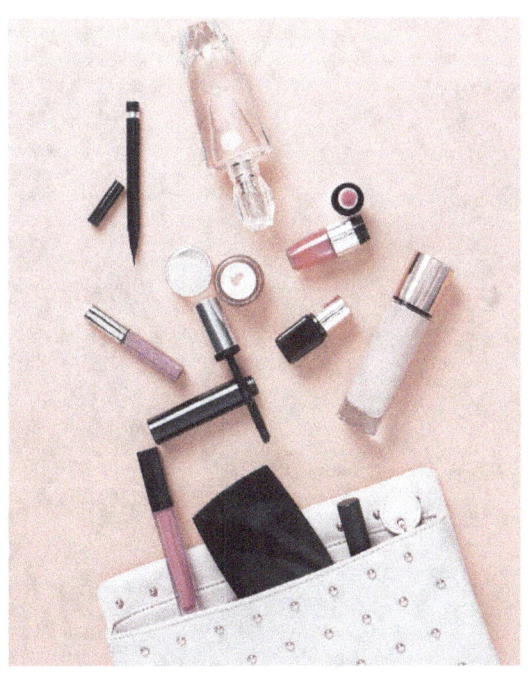

Endocrine Disrupting Chemicals do exactly that, for example most commonly they mimic Estrogen, this **artificial Estrogen then knocks our other Hormones out of Balance** like calming, mood soothing Progesterone and therefore can be seen with symptoms like increased Anxiety or Low Mood.

Since our Hormones are nothing other than chemical secretions by our endocrine glands. Such as our thyroid, pancreas, pituitary, and so on. **They control the functions of all the important organs in the body**

Now before you start to freak out or panic, like I did too when I first discovered this. Knowledge is power and once you know what to look out for you are better informed and so the opportunity to choose to be be better protected.

This doesn't mean I'm telling you to immediately ditch all of your Personal Care Products. This Guide is titled how to Look good and Feel Better- there are ways to deal with this dilemma. Besides everyone is going to react differently to their level of exposure. What I'm advocating is to do your own due diligence. What actually is in the Ingredients of the Products you are using? You can do your own research at the EWG.com Website. What I did was replace my products with Clean Beauty alternatives. Its no wonder Clean Beauty is one of the fastest growing industries, since once you know you are actually spritzing yourself in Toxic Pheromones- mainstream Perfume looses its appeal. But now you can get really good replicates that are made with 'Hormone Friendly' Essential Oils from someone like EDEN . Ingestible Beauty Supplements are also a great alternative in the next chapter we will find more about how they work.

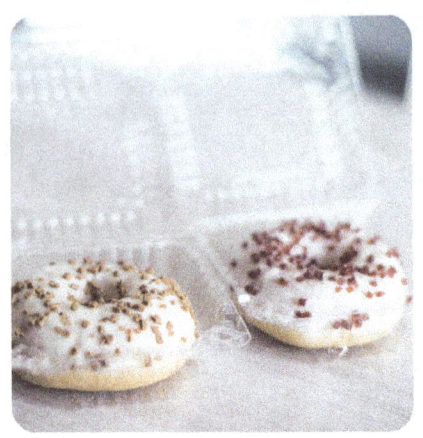 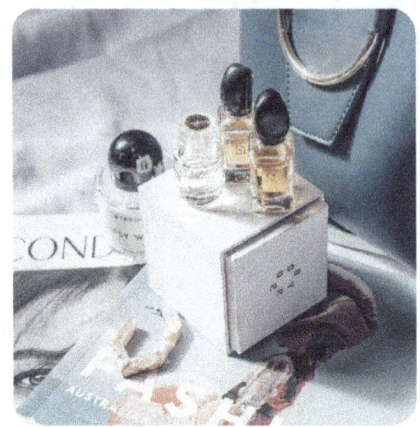 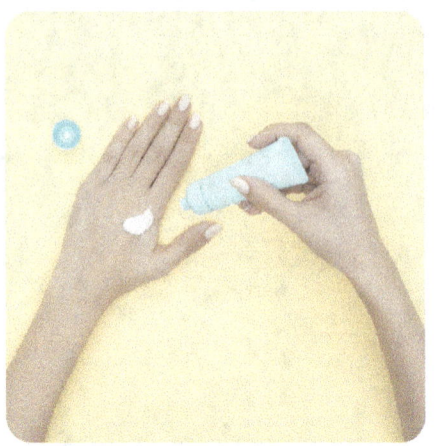

Endocrine Disrupting Chemicals and where they are found!

Very few people are aware of just how many Endocrine Disrupting Chemicals (EDC) are in the household products they use everyday.

The concerning statistics are that the increasing exposure to EDCs over the past 20 years appear responsible for the growing number of people with Infertility, Diabetes, early onset of Puberty in Girls and early Menopause in Women, Cancer, Birth defects, and Neurobehavioral disorders, according to a statement issued by the Endocrine Society and IPEN (International Pollutants Elimination Network)

Yes it is a big deal! but we don't need to Stress, we can easily protect ourselves once we know this information.
But really please don't Stress, we can't remove every Toxin in our environment but studies show by using this information to reduce your exposure this is enough to have a positive impact on our natural Hormone levels

Where are EDCs mainly found ?
-Plastics
- Meat and foods (non organic)
-Sugar
- Make up
- Fragrances
-Household Cleaning Products

Yes that is a lot of products!
Mainly look out for parabens, BPA , Sulphates, Pesticides , Flame retardants, unfortunately most Plastics release Estrogenic Chemicals

How to reduce your own exposure

-Choose natural whole healthy foods (organic where possible)
-Reduce Sugar
-Reduce Toxins
-Avoid Plastic Packaging
-Reducing Stress
-Go for clean beauty and cosmetics

see the Endocrine Society's website for a full list and the 'THINK DIRTY 'APP

Hormone Imbalance is our body calling for help

80% of us experience Hormone Imbalance at some stage in our lives. Becoming aware of the impact of Hormonal Imbalances is the first step towards increasing your chances of a Happier, Healthier Life. Many Women feel like they just need to carry on putting up with unpleasant side affects without realising most of which can be fully treated Naturally with the right help once you know.

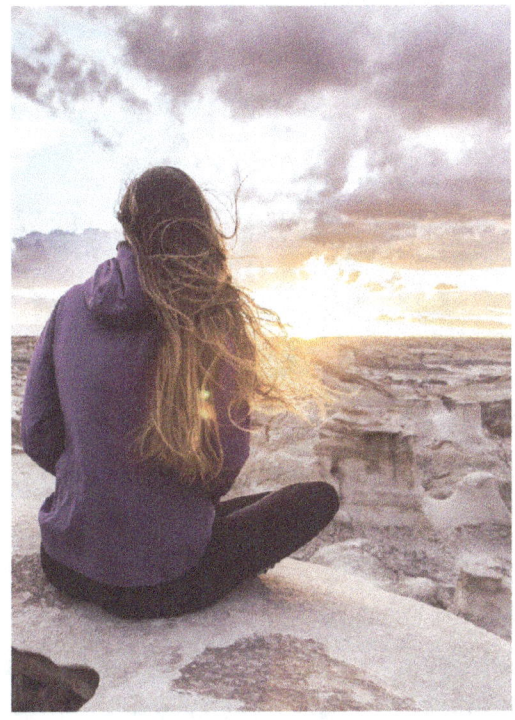

Examples of why balance is important:

 Progesterone regulates other Hormone levels which is why it's so important to be in Balance. Low Progesterone is the most common imbalance, it is mainly caused by Artificial Estrogen from Endocrine Disruptors. This is a big deal since it Affects: Mood, Weight, Fertility, Health, Immunity *the list goes on..*

 High Estrogen/ Estrogen dominance then causes even lower Progesterone levels. We will go into why this matters further on in the Guide.

 Progesterone is needed for regular Ovulation and a Healthy shedding of Uterus lining (Period) for Healthy Cycles and to prevent further imbalance and even protection of certain Cancers from un-apposed Estrogen levels. Progesterone is also needed for a Pregnancy to continue! A Major factor in infertility.

Estrogen is not the Enemy Low Estrogen can also be a problem in fact artificial Estrogen mimickers can not only cause Dominance but can also cause low 'Natural' Estrogen levels. Estrogen deficiency is less common than Dominance this is caused by too much depletion in the Body and can be seen with Headache ands Light Periods.

 High Testosterone - in Women can affect the Balance of other Hormones such as Insulin, Blood sugar levels, Egg quality, Hair and Acne

 Oestrogen dominance happens when Progesterone levels drop too low. Oestrogen is needed for Egg quality

 Ongoing Stress= High cortisol- when cortisol levels spike it blocks Progesterone receptors and limits the activity of Progesterone

PROTECTING THE NATURAL BALANCE IS THE KEY!

Could you be one of the Many Women with an Inositol Deficiency?

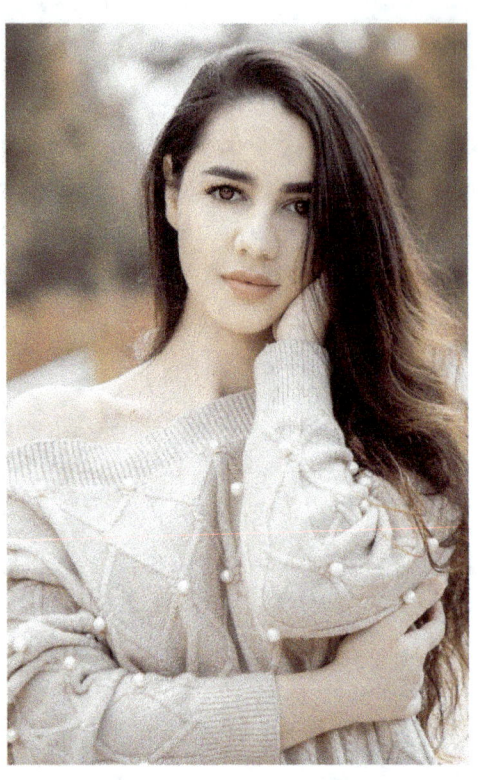

Although Inositol is naturally produced in the Body, some Women have been found to have a defect in how they metabolise it, resulting in Nutritional deficiencies and Hormone Imbalances. Some of the more obvious symptoms are Anxiety, Weight gain and Imbalanced Blood Sugars. And difficulty loosing Weight.

Many Women have found that this is where Supplementing with Myo-Inositol can help to bridge the gap. One of the main symptoms of Hormone Imbalance affects the Gut Health and also causes Sugar Cravings. People with low levels of Myo Inositol in their Body have been found to suffer from Anxiety. Myo Inositol supplementation is believed to help stimulate the production of 'Feel Good' Hormones Serotonin and Dopamine.

Myo-Inositol has been shown to help with Sugar Cravings and can help Balance Blood Sugars and Weight loss as it acts as an Insulin Sensitizer.
So it is involved in the way that Glucose is managed in the body (in non Diabetic Women). Which helps to support and can potentially reduce the risk of developing Insulin Resistance which can lead to further Health Issues such as Metabolic Syndrome.
Myo-Inositol is used as a Safe and Natural alternative choice to Metformin by many Women with PCOS. Since it is a Nutraceutical derived from Foods but can not always be obtained by diet alone. My Myo Plan is readily converted into the highly absorbable Myo-Inositol type. Results can be seen within Weeks.

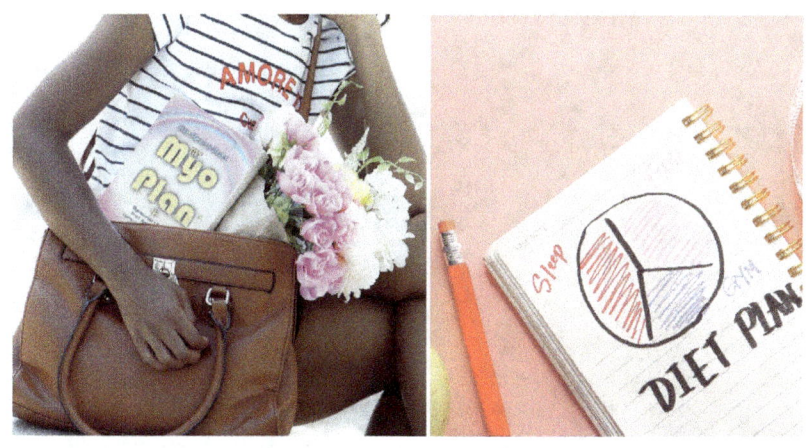

Be your own Health Advocate!

Before taking any Supplement we recommend you do your own research. Studies have shown Myo-Inositol can help to lower levels of Androgen's helping to support and **rebalance other Hormones in the Body.**
Such as Progesterone which is necessary for restoring regular Menstrual Cycles. This can also **aid Fertility by stimulating Ovulation, to help maintain an ongoing Healthy Hormone Balance.**
Un-apposed Estrogen from not Ovulating regularly causes a whole host of Health issues the biggest is a higher risk of developing Cancer. So rest assured that you can now support your Natural Balance.

Also Myo-Inositol help **to reduce the development of Acne.** Because lowering Androgen's can decrease the Oil in the Skin. My Myo Plan + has added **Antioxidants that go straight to the Cell. Going further as an internal Beauty supplement nourishing your Skin, Hair and Hormones.**

The only Nutraceutical Brand that we recommend is My Myo Plan, since it was created by our Hormone Health & Nutrition Coach Kerry Goodliffe and one of the only Brands to contain Purely The
Myo-Inositol and Antioxidant Formula instead of the D-Chiro type. Since not everyone suits the standard 40:1 ratio in most brands we offer the pure Myo type you can read more on in the Clinical Research Trials.. We have a special discount for our readers go to HormoneHealthBliss.com

What is Poly Cystic Ovary Syndrome? and why you need to know

Poly Cystic Ovary Syndrome is one of the most underdiagnosed and misunderstood Female Health conditions, even though around 10-15% of Women live with this. The misconception is you need Cysts to be diagnosed but this is outdated-its more to do with the FSH and LH ratio and high Androgen and Insulin levels. Insulin Resistance is a major symptom and Sugar Cravings can be a sign of this.

PCOS is commonly diagnosed after Infertility or recurrent Miscarriage as it is one of the leading causes.
In particular high levels of Follicle Stimulating Hormone (FSH) can reduce the likelihood of conception and healthy mature eggs from being released at the right time since to be healthy they need time to mature to undergo the Fertilization process and Thrive later down the line.

Another issue for PCOS: Low levels of Luteinizing Hormone (LH). This would be what stimulates the ovaries to release an egg and start producing Progesterone, which is needed for the Fertilised Egg to Embed in the Womb and also the Pregnancy to continue. So both FSH and LH need to be at the right levels.

Why are high FSH levels a problem?- they can be an indicator of how many eggs you have left in your ovaries and if it is high, the harder your body has to work to mature the egg for ovulation.

PCOS not only affects Fertility it is a Metabolic Disorder and requires intervention to prevent Health issues like Diabetes, Heart Disease High Blood Pressure ect. But fear not with the right Treatment and Help your Health can be optimised contact me for details of my PCOS Powerplan at mymyoplan@gmail.com

Common Symptoms of Hormone Imbalance with PCOS

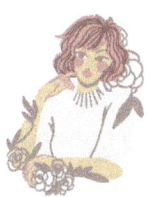

- Imbalanced blood sugars
- Cravings for sweet and carbohydrate foods
- Headaches
- Irregular periods
- Lack of periods
- Lack of ovulation
- Heavy painful periods
- Acne

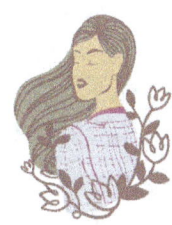

- Hirsutism
- Mood swings
- Hair on abdomen and or nipples and face
- Low sex drive or high sex drive
- Anxiety
- Depression
- Headaches
- If the time from ovulation to period is either too long or too short
- FSH or LH imbalance

What you can do- Speak to your doctor about tests for PCOS and request your FSH and LH Level ratios to be checked.

They should offer you Insulin resistance tests but if not also request these, the most common tests for insulin levels are the fasting tests and the glucose fasting test where you are given a sugary drink and then tested.

Thyroid Issues

Another major Health concern is from Undiagnosed thyroid dysfunction. Not only can make it difficult to
Loose Weight and affects the Metabolism. The Thyroid is also responsible for Energy and regulating body temperature. An imbalance can lead to further Health Issues.

Symptoms:

Underactive Thyroid
Tired
Weight gain
Sensitive to cold
Irregular periods
Depression
Muscle aches
Cramps and weakness

Overactive Thyroid
Nervous
Restless
Anxious
Neck swelling
Irritability
Muscle weakness
Mood swings
Sensitive to heat
Hyperactivity
Weight loss

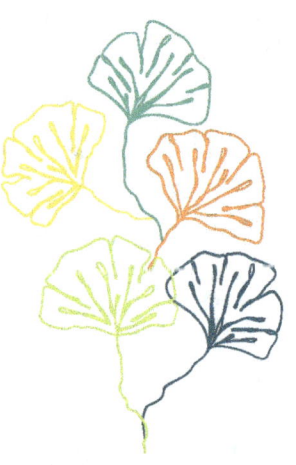

Ask for a full thyroid function test f you want to investigate further. Both types can be treated with medication.
A Hormone Healthy Eating Plan such as discussed later in this Guide will help to support the Thyroid

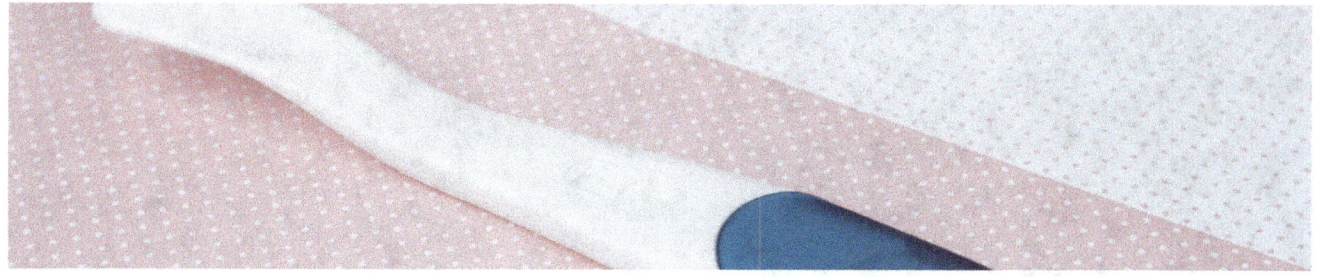

Periods and Ovulation

Whether you are trying to conceive or not our Cycle Health is important for our overall Health. Our Period is recognised as the 5th Vital Sign and our Bodies way of communicating with us.

A Healthy Menstrual Cycle is needed to have the right balance of Hormones to be able to Ovulate

Causes of lack of Menstruation and or Ovulation:

Stress
Undereating
Over exercise
Anorexia
Overweight
PCOS
Endometriosis
Medication
Emotional/ Mental Block
Imbalanced Hormones

If you are not TTC (Trying to Conceive) go to the next page.
If you are TTC and using Ovulation prediction tests?
You could be getting a 'false' positive! Clinical studies have reported this widely for decades! Especially for conditions such as PCOS where your LH levels will be higher at other points in the month not just around Ovulation.
I also find women tell me that Ovulation prediction tests are also stress inducing for them, which in itself can hinder Ovulation from happening.

And If, like many women are beating yourself up for infertility and have told yourself a story of it being your fault, you should free yourself from this thought. It won't help to think that it would have been anything you did. As the type of person to even be reading this book you have already shown that you want to do the best you can for your reproductive health I have a whole section coming up on TTC and another Planner Guide focused purely on how to 'Get Pregnant Faster' . Email me at mymyoplan@gmail.com for a Free copy.

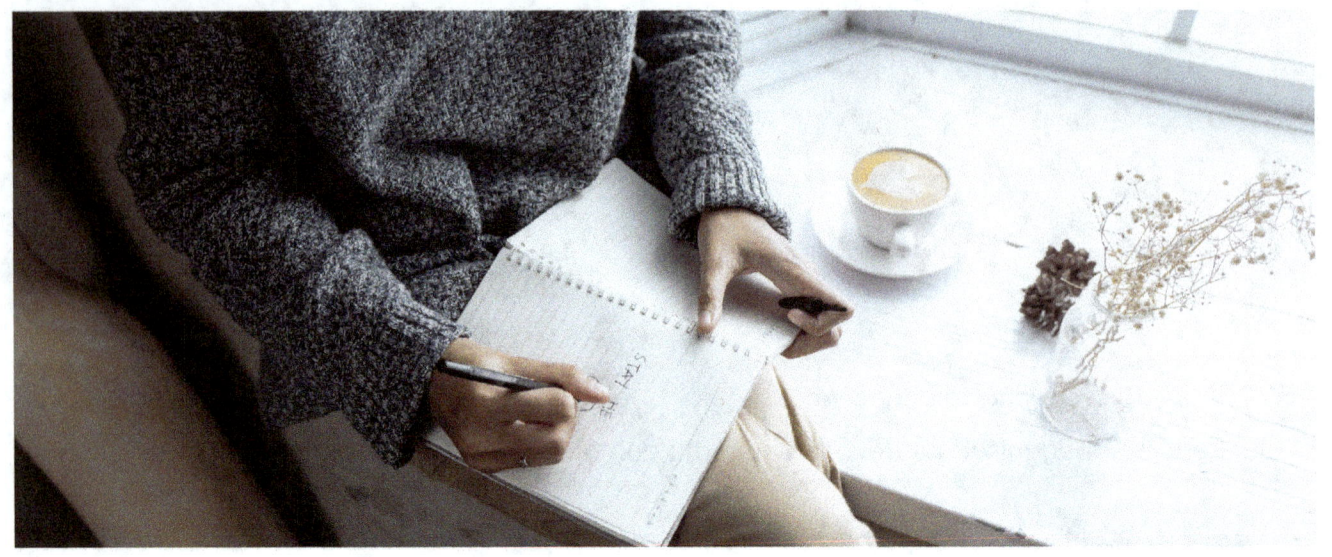

Low Progesterone

We have seen already in this guide that Stress, EDC's, Processed Foods and a Unhealthy Diet can cause Low Progesterone- and other Hormones to become Imbalanced the main chronic causes otherwise are Thyroid disorders, and PCOS can cause irregular or lack of ovulation which would lead to Low Progesterone levels. The reasons for low Progesterone needs to be diagnosed and treated rather than only supplementing with progesterone alone since there can be several underlying causes.

The reason why we are focusing on Low Progesterone is it is most common cause is due to Estrogen dominance, since it will cause a Progesterone/Estrogen imbalance this is becoming an increasingly prevalent issue for women today since it is caused from Endocrine disrupting Chemicals or an accumulation of these in our environment. EDCs are everywhere let's get one step ahead by learning how to avoid them.

If you suspect you have low Progesterone get a blood test on day 21 of your cycle or if your cycle is longer or shorter liaise with your medical team on when would be best for you personally. So if you have a 35 day cycle you'll want to test on day 28 or day 14 if you have a 21 day cycle generally!.

Following a 'Hormone Healthy Foods' plan in this Guide will also help you reduce Inflammation the major factor behind Hormone and Metabolic Health! . This eating plan is also for Thyroid and pre-conception support as it is based on Mediterranean and Low GI foods - with a few extra tweaks to further support egg and sperm health!.

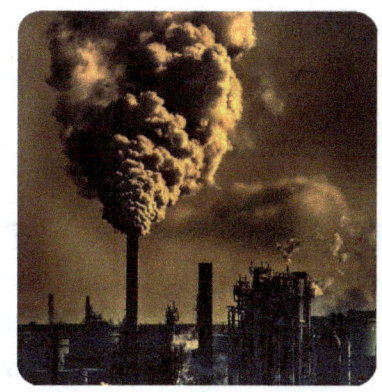

AIR POLLUTION AND HOW IT AFFECTS THE ENDOCRINE SYSTEM

Daily exposure to pollution is another form of Endocrine disruption and has been associated with irregular cycles, reduced rates of fertility ect since the pollutants enter our bodies they trick the normal functioning of our Hormones: increasing the production of certain Hormones like cortisol and reducing others.

What can you do to reduce your risk

- **Check air quality in your area http://airnow.gov**
- **Avoid driving, exercising or walking in high traffic areas from roads, buses or trains**
- **Avoid outdoor exercise if pollution levels are high**
- **Wear a mask if you have to commute**
- **Choose routes that limit your time sat in traffic**
- **Blow your nose when you get to work (after your commute and when you get home) especially in hayfever season**
- **Avoid polluted streets – take a diversion if you can**
- **Check air pollution apps**
- **Avoid rush hour exercise**
- **Eat a healthy diet!**

There is a growing amount of research to say what we eat may help to mitigate the harmful effects of air pollution. This study was based on Mediterranean style eating and conducted by New York University's School of Medicine. The study states that although pollution causes oxidation in the body if you have enough antioxidants in your body then they can help to neutralise it! Also there are so many great alternatives nowadays and the Endocrine Society's website is a great resource to check your products' toxic load.

Hormone Friendly Foods
STRATEGY

Follow a healthy, and low glycemic index Mediterranean type diet

According to the studies, a healthy diet and good lifestyle choices results in a lower risk of Hormone Imbalances, Infertility and Ovulatory disorder compared to Women who eat unhealthy and packaged foods, which have a high content of endocrine disrupting chemicals.

The best type of diet to follow for ultimate health by the WHO World Health Organisation was voted the Mediterranean and I have also adapted this with foods with low GI index. Such as non startchy vegetables, legumes, fresh fruits, oatmeal, and quinoa.

In the pre-ovulation phase (ideally 90 days prior to conceiving), a well-balanced sugar intake will maintain the blood sugar and insulin levels. This will also help to prevent the occurrence of gestational diabetes during pregnancy and improve the body's metabolism.

Natural fertility will significantly increase if processed foods high in carbohydrates are avoided. This includes foods such as bread, pasta, cookies, and other packaged foods. It will limit the intake of EDC and has shown beneficial results in women who are trying to conceive and have PCOS (Polycystic Ovarian Syndrome)

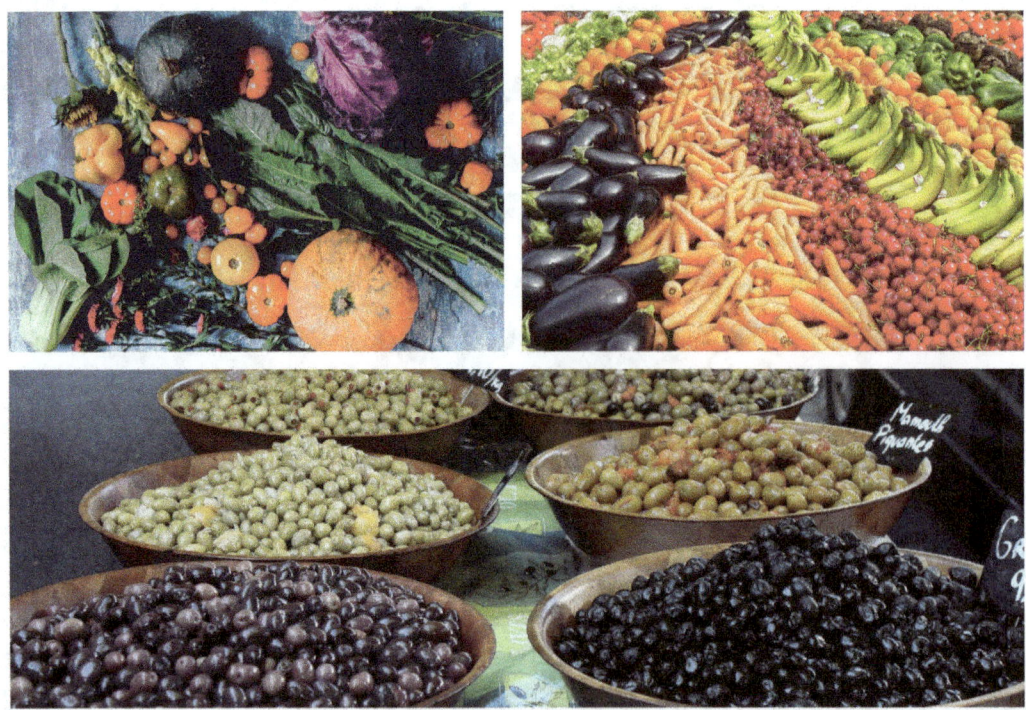

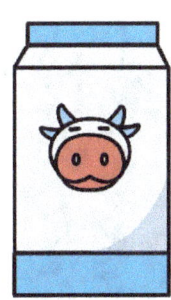

GO WITH YOUR GUT

Gut Instinct

Another major factor in having a healthy hormone balance is how your gut can work with you or against you for good overall health. Without a healthy microbiome estrogen metabolism and function can become impaired and can lead to health consequences such as;

Estrogen dominance can lead to Sugar cravings increasing inflammation and impacting Gut Health and can be seen in:

-Endometriosis
-PCOS
-Endometrial hyperplasia
-Infertility
-Pregnancy complications
-And many more longer term Health issues
if left untreated
-An imbalanced gut can also be a sign of Thyroid issues

Estrogen is not the Enemy Low Estrogen is also an issue. Balance is key!

SUPPORT THE GUT BY SUPPORTING THE LIVER!
EAT YOUR GREENS
ADD :FIBRE
MACA ROOT
DIM (DIINDOLYLMETHANE)
PROBIOTICS
MYO INOSITOL
AVOIDING EDC'S, PECTICIDES & SUGAR
AVOID ARFTIFICIAL SOY PRODUCTS AND PROCESSED FOODS IN GENERAL

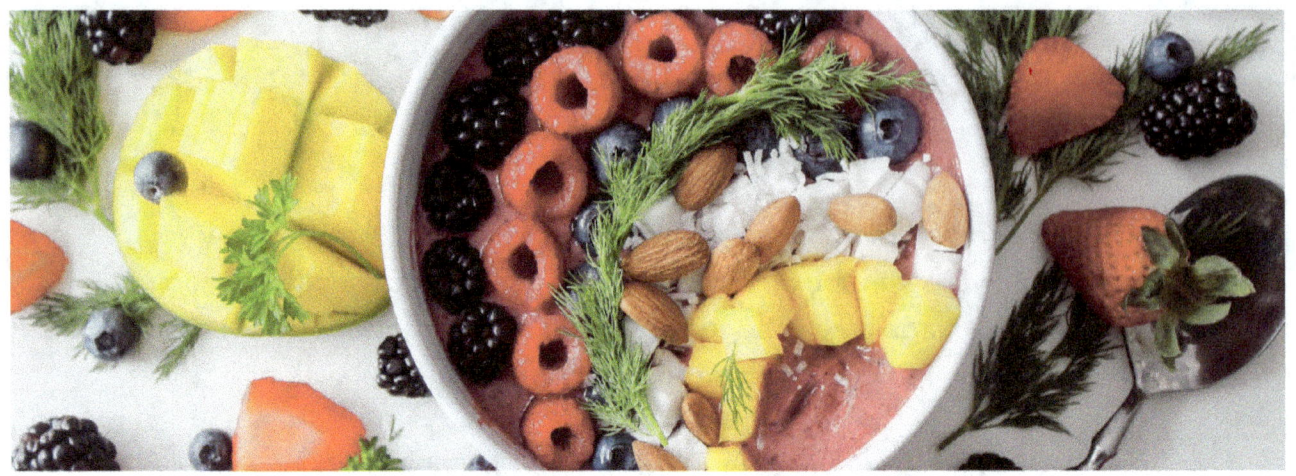

Nourish yourself

Focus on eating immune boosting foods, rich in vegetables and fruits like, spinach, papaya, apple, pomegranate, broccoli, cauliflower, cabbage, quinoa, amaranth, barley and cooking with Coconut Oil. These nutrients provide fibers, essential micronutrients, vitamins, iron, calcium, essential fatty acids, antioxidants and flavonoids that boost immune system and decrease toxic elements.

Avoid packaged foods as they disrupt the endocrine system balance and impair overall health. Research has shown that women who have a habit of eating processed foods, find it difficult to conceive naturally. Infertility increases when a diet has more starchy foods, and caffeine intake is high. Studies have mentioned that intake of stimulants spikes up estrogen levels due to increased activity of the adrenal glands.

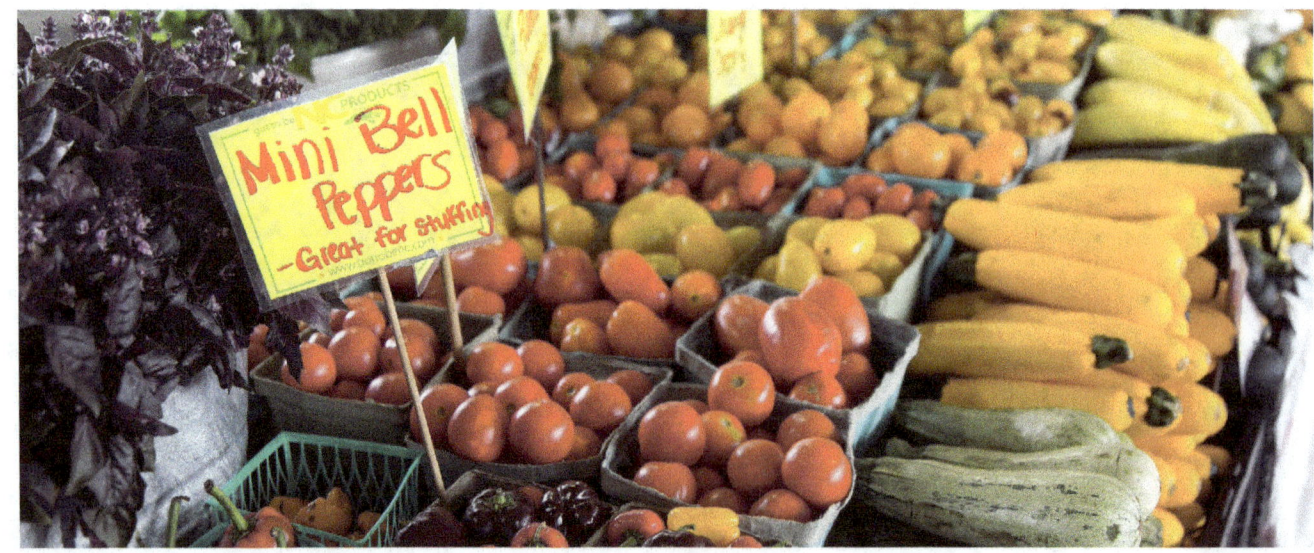

Foods to Avoid

Limit – starchy white carbs which include:

- Anything made from flour
- Rice (white)
- Potatoes
- Bread (worst is white and bagels)
- Foods containing sugar–
- All sugars
- Products containing fructose and corn syrup – without the fruit!
- Potato chips
- Pasta
- Ice cream
- Soda/fizzy drinks– even sugar free
- Fast food
- Pizza
- Cereal
- Instant processed oats

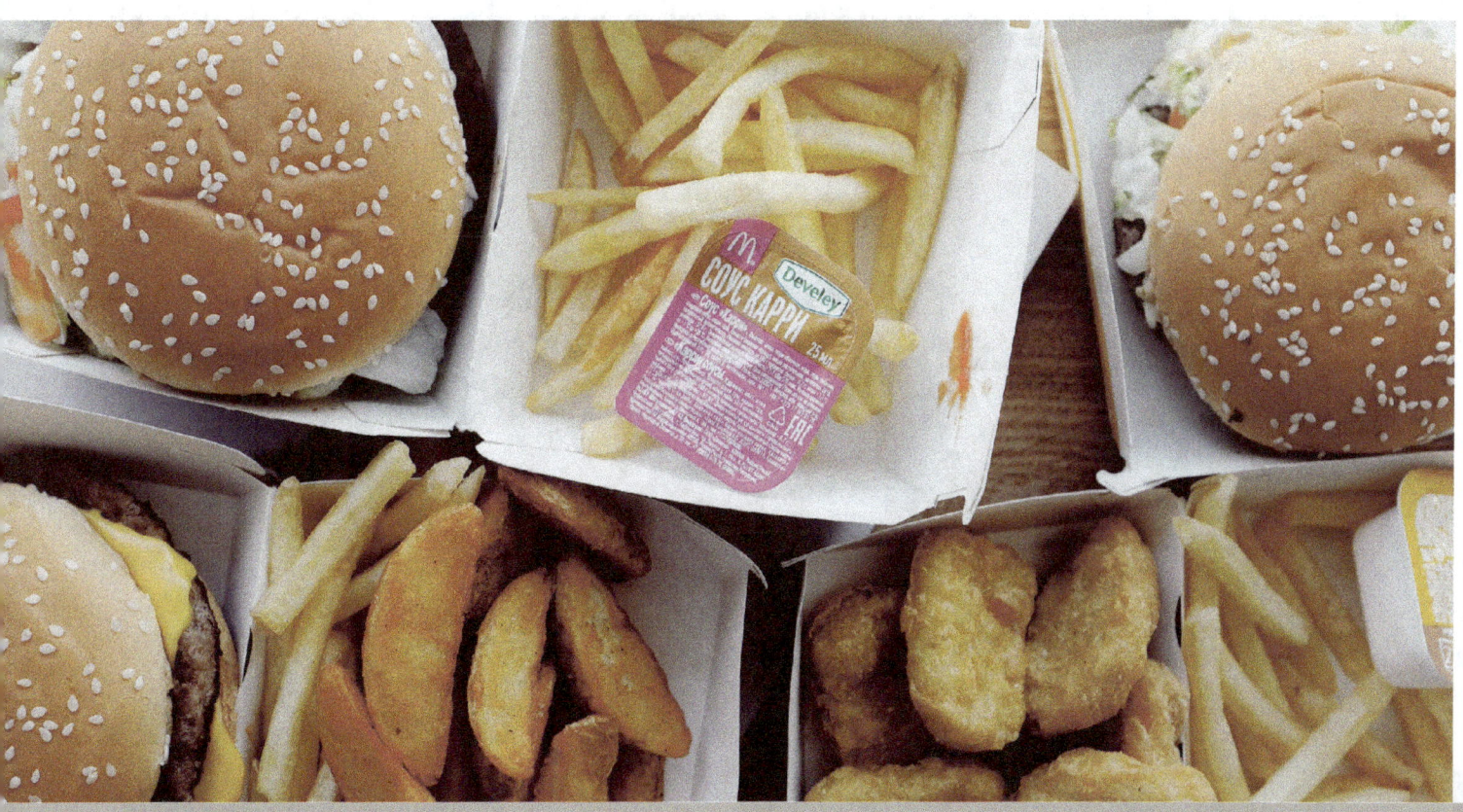

Foods to Eat More of

Slow Release Carbs:

- Vegetables <u>no limit</u> – fill up and fall in love with them!
- Berries and lower sugar fruits (see list)
- Quinoa
- Beans
- Seeds
- Brown rice
- Buckwheat
- Nuts
- Fish
- High fiber foods
- Unrefined whole grains
- Bran cereal
- Wholemeal spaghetti
- Lentils
- Chickpeas
- Wholemeal couscous
- Use olive oil and coconut oil instead of any other types of fats

and 'clean' protein! such as Organic. Since farmed meats and fish raised on an unnatural diet that is focused on producing quantity not quality may contain high levels of hormones, antibiotics, PCBs, and mercury. These are also endocrine-disrupting chemicals (EDCs) – If you are vegan still get your protein but avoid soya- otherwise go for organic lower saturated fat types of meat and cheese if possible. Ideally focus on non meat varieties.

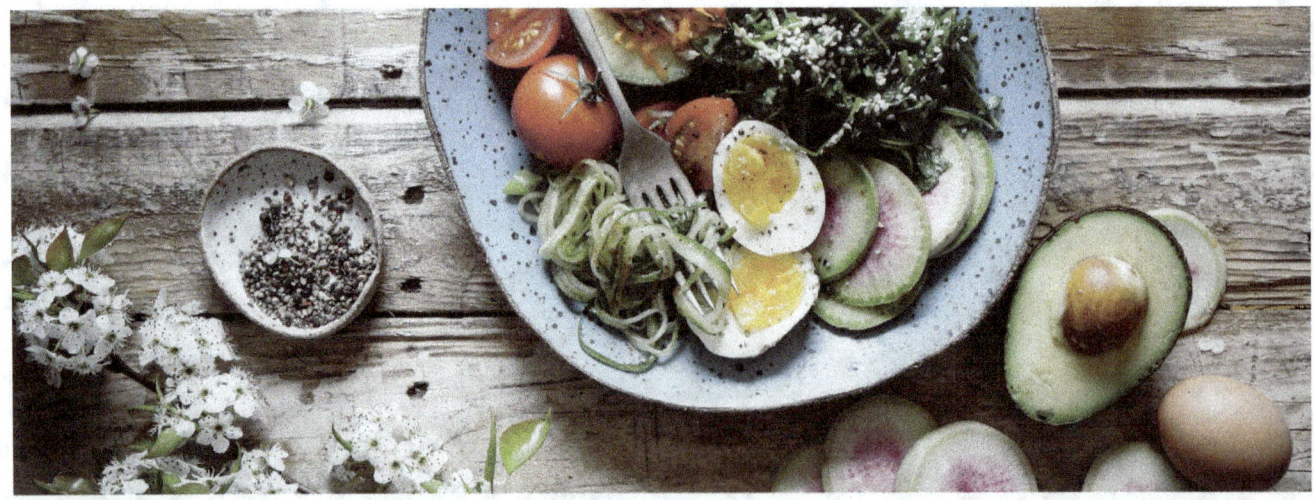

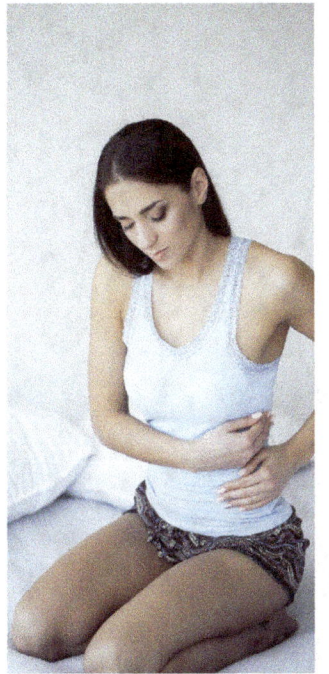
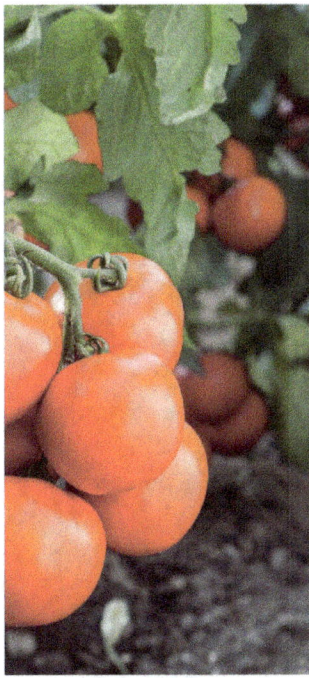

Could eliminating Tomato change everything for you?

Not all Fruits and Vegetables are equal coming up we go through the Sugar level lists but see below the 'harmless' Tomato is actually in the Nightshade category these seem to affect some people especially those with autoimmune diseases in particular Crohn's and Irritable Bowel Disease or Leaky Gut people with these Health Issues have eliminated Nightshades from their diets and found an improvement in their symptoms This is not that surprising since some of the other plants and vegetables in the Nightshade family are actually Poisonous such as Belladonna. People that are sensitive to Nightshade are also likely to have Fructose intolerance and notice the biggest change in their symptoms cutting from back on Sugars and Sweeteners.

Common Nightshade Vegetables:

- Eggplants
- Peppers
- Tabacco
- Tomatillos
- Tomatoes

The 1 Cup Comparison of Fruit Sugar Levels

Higher Sugar- Eat sparingly:

- Raisins
- Cranberries (dried)
- Apricots (dried)
- Peaches (dried)
- Prunes
- Dates
- Grapes
- Kiwi
- Pineapple
- Papaya
- Persimmons
- Banana (cooked or over ripe)
- Jackfruit
- Pomegranate (juice)
- Pear
- Orange (juice)
- Most canned fruits especially in syrup other than the natural juice

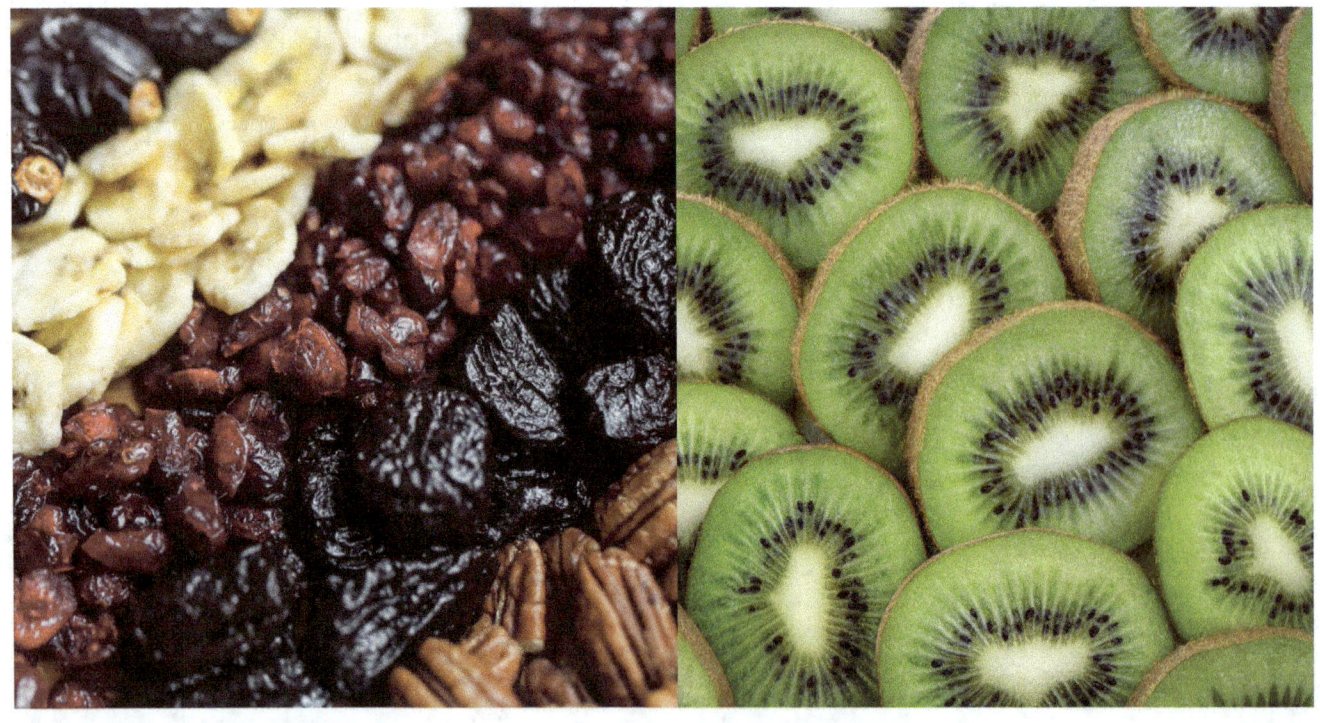

The 1 Cup Comparison of Fruit Sugar Levels

Medium Sugar:

- Mango
- Orange
- Apple
- Cherries
- Banana (less ripe)

These lists are not exhaustive but for your quick reference it gives you a general guide you can obtain full GI Lists online although you will find some
confliction on ratings the most trustworthy are from the American Diabetes Association

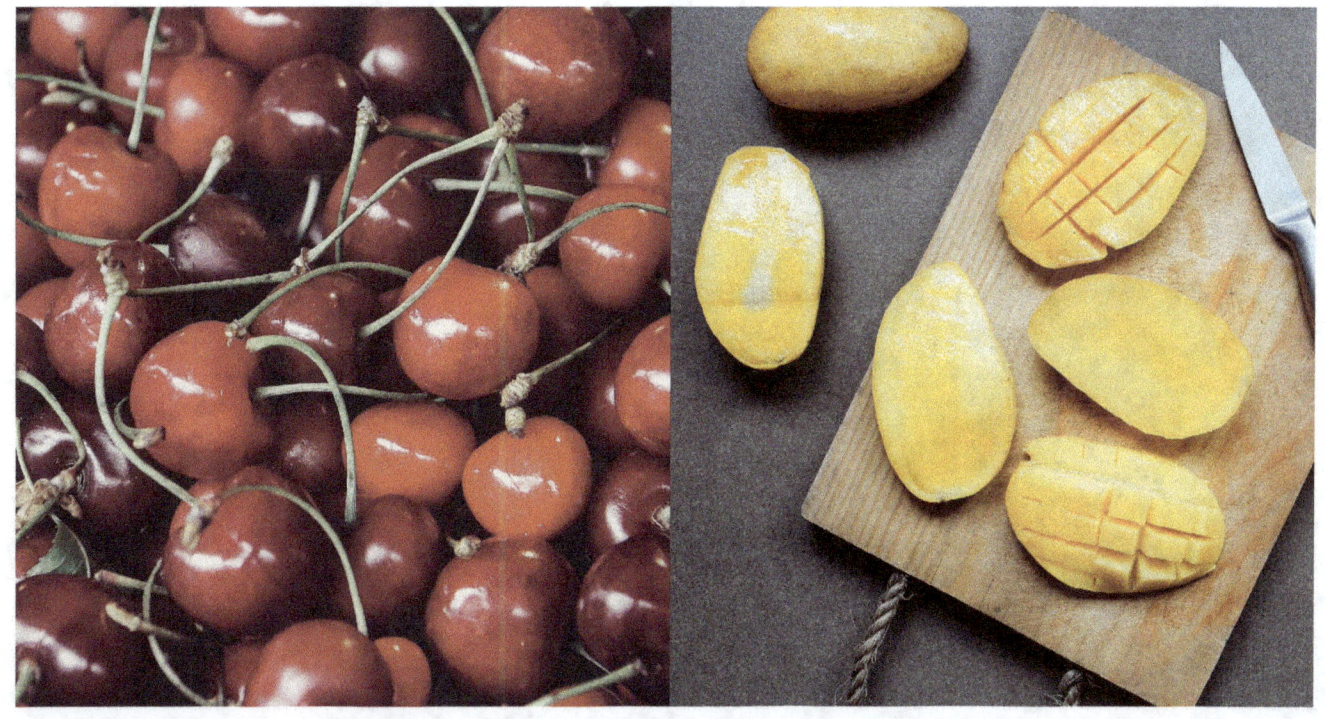

The 1 Cup Comparison of Fruit Sugar Levels

Lower Sugar:

- Most Berries
- Strawberries
- Blueberries
- Peach
- Raspberries
- Grapefruit
- Apricots (fresh)
- Clementine
- Lime (juice)
- Lemon
- Nectarines
- Peaches (yellow)
- Cantaloupe
- Blackberries

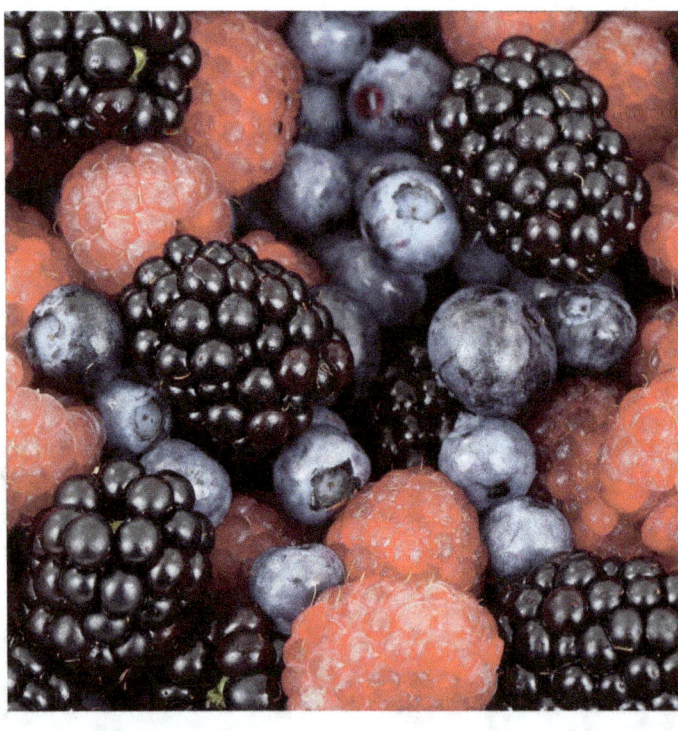
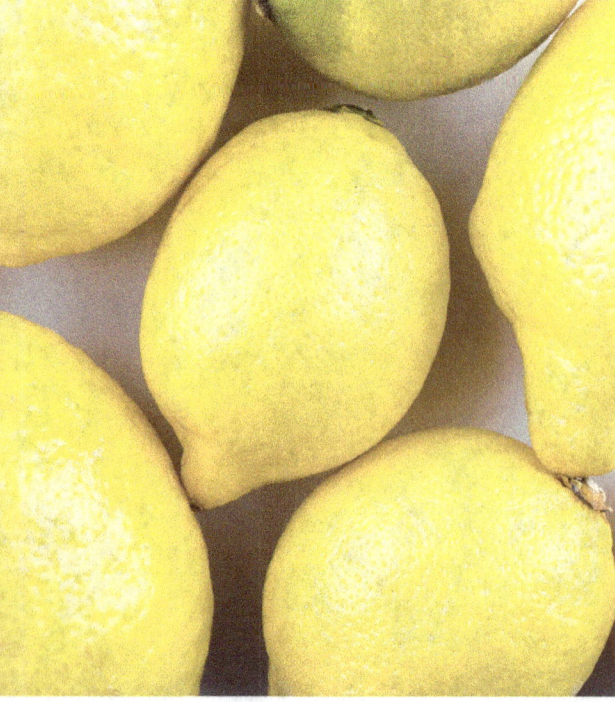

FOODS THAT ARE GOOD FOR BALANCING HORMONES AND ANTI-INFLAMMATORY:

This is not a diet, it is a long term healthy eating lifestyle plan so it is not focused on what you need to avoid and/or counting calories instead place your focus on getting more of the foods you can have and are recommended by filling up on vegetables first.
Try not to think of foods as good and bad but ask yourself the question - Will this be nourishing for my body?

Healthy Hormone fuel:

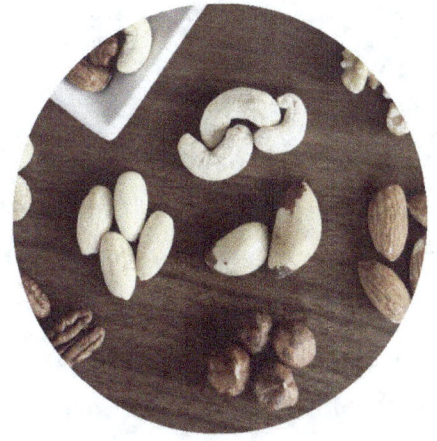

Leafy Greens

Broccoli

Avocado

Beans

Chia Seeds

Sunflower Seeds

Seasame seeds

Pumpkin Seeds

Flax Seeds

Almonds

Walnuts

Olives

Tumeric

Lentils

Blueberries

Blackberries

Dark Chocolate

Ginger Root

Coconut

Raw

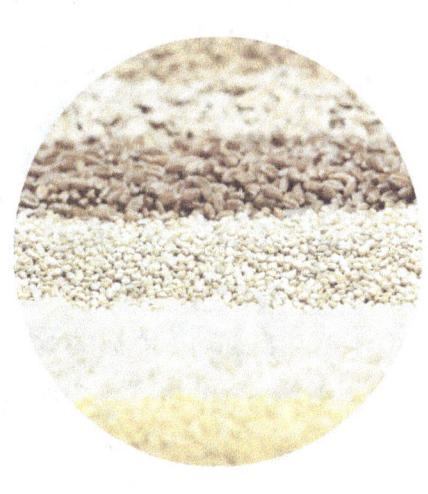

Making it Easier to Live a Lower Sugar Lifestyle long term

The following information about Sugar is to help reframe your existing knowledge and association with Sugar and Sweetners. The most important part of keeping up a long term Healthy Eating Plan is to **change our Psychological responses and beliefs** for a long time we have been associating Sugary foods as pure pleasure and something we 'deserve' as a way to cheer ourselves up ironically instead of celebrating 'Life prolonging Healthy Foods'. I'm not being a kill joy. Infact my whole aim is to **find Healthier Sweet tasting alternatives to give people better options** and be more likely to stick to lower sugar living for longer. As I know where you may come up against challenges. Since **I've been living this way for over 15 years and reversed my Insulin Resistant PCOS**, so I know its entirely possible and something I teach others to do with my Courses and Coaching. If you would like extra help breaking up with Sugar I even have a Hypnosis recording on cutting down the cravings for good. in the three step program 'Low Sugar Living- Combat Cravings the easy way'!. details to follow.

But first I have to ask you are you really ready for this? Because its not as much a physical challenge as a mental and emotional one, its why I do Mindset support coaching along with the combat cravings package.
Are you willing to face the facts that you can't turn your back on? They say we only regret the things we don't do in Life. Will you look back and kick yourself if you don't make the changes that you know deep down will make you Happier Healthier and give you back the body of your Youth? What more motivation could you have apart from asking you to think about who else will benefit? Loved ones, Children, Friends and Relatives will all see the change in you and either secretly or openly admire you for making these changes for your Health and Life.

I'm with you, I live this way. I have no other choice. And I love it. Come with me lets do this!

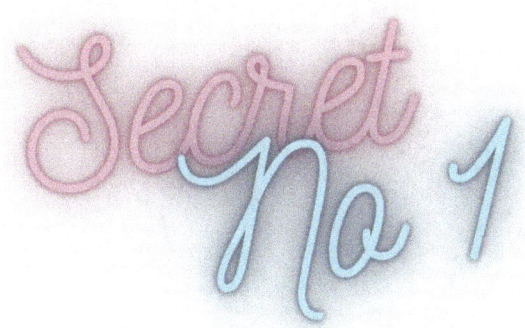

How to help Curb the Cravings :
By Eating Chocolate!

According to the Studies, eating a small amount – 1 or 2 Squares per day of high quality dark chocolate in the morning may help stabilize your blood sugar levels by limiting your sweet cravings. Be warned that not all Chocolate is created equally. It needs to be the lower Sugar Dark type which can also have Gut Health and Antioxidant Benefits. Beware of anything lower than 80% Cocoa or with added Sugar or Sweeteners like Fructose and Dark Chocolate contains Caffeine. Unfortunately there are so many 'bad for you bars' out there it can be confusing. For that reason we filtered and sifted the market and found The Beauty Bar: an Organic, Vegan Sugar Free Brand that is one of the few Sweetened with Monk Fruit one of the most Natural and safe Sugar Alternatives. It also has added Collagen and other Beauty benefits our Nutrtionist was so impressed by the Health Boosting Ingredients It is why we use them in our 'Lower Sugar Life-Combat Chocolate Cravings the Easy way Plan which combines:
- A Daily Hypnotherapy 'Sugar Craving control' recording
-Sugar Craving Coaching on how to retrain and reframe your attitude to Chocolate
-A months Supply of Hormone Supportive and Anti Craving Supplement My Myo Plan
-The Beauty Bar Chocolate to use in this Training package to Detox your Sugar Sensitivity and Reset your Gut Health to help the Cravings long term!
Message; mymyoplan@gmail.com to join the next intake!

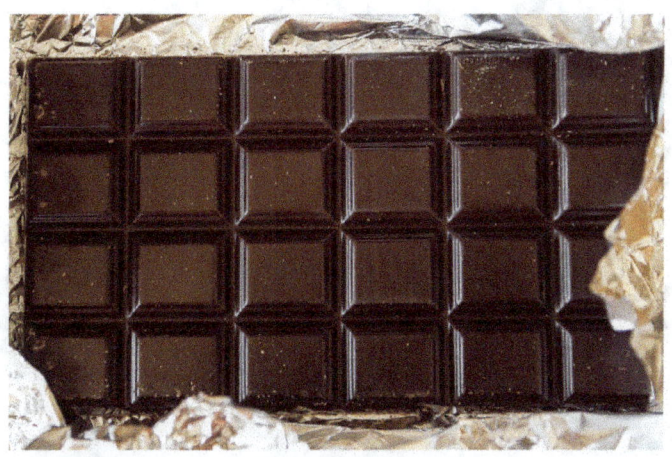

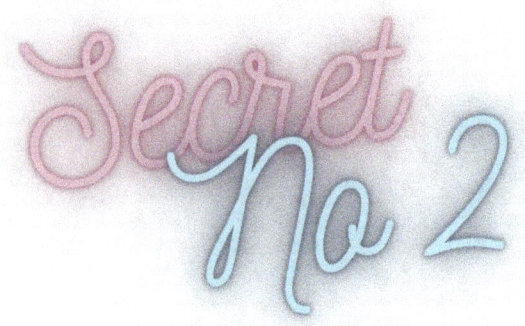

A Green Smoothie a day keeps the Cravings at bay!

How to Stay Full through the day and get your Veggies in!. Make up 1 large glass of at least 3 part Veg to 1 part Fruit. Green Smoothie. Add A Non Dairy Milk like Coconut or Almond and a Whey or Pea based Protein Powder. It is a great way to get your Fibre in, to make up for if you don't get your plate filled with the recommended daily Veg count!. Since Fibre in Fruits and Vegetables is what we need to help flush out excess Estrogen out of our system for Healthier Hormones.

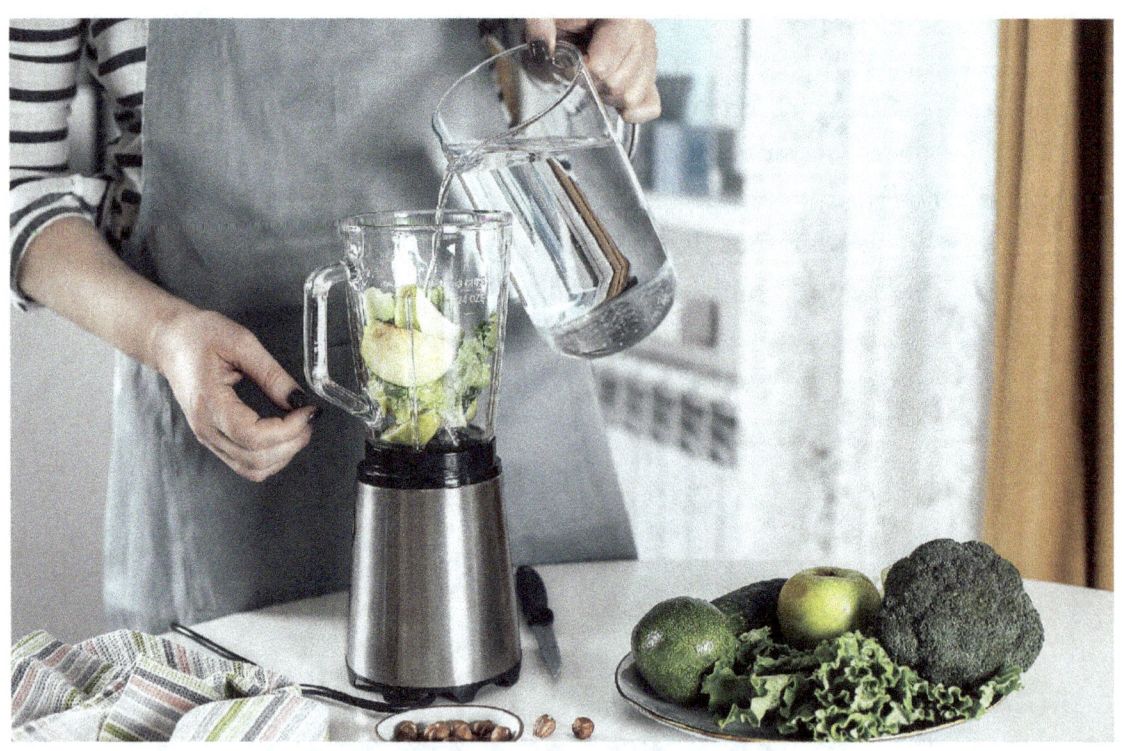

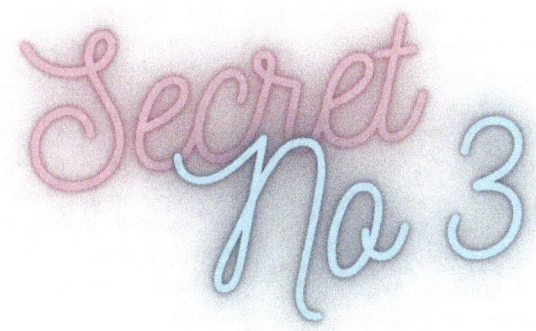

Secret
No 3

10 minutes a Day of Walking or gentle Exercise will stimulate your Metabolism and help stabalize Blood Sugars leading to less Cravings

It may not be that surprising for you to learn that the vast majority of fitness research is based on A Mans fitness profile rather than a Women's. Or caters to the unique Hormonal differences of being A Female, and how to work with the different Hormones. Consider that for a minute. You have been following advice and doing programs built on research that was done on men, NOT women. Not only that, but these men were mainly between 18-20 years old. So Its worth learning which types of exercise is best for your Unique Hormones and at which point is best to suit your Cycle needs. We are starting a Programme shortly working with a Well known Fitness Trainer that is going to be designed to support all Women's Unique Hormone needs and Cycle's. If you would like to be added to the waiting list for this email: kerry.healthplan@gmail.com

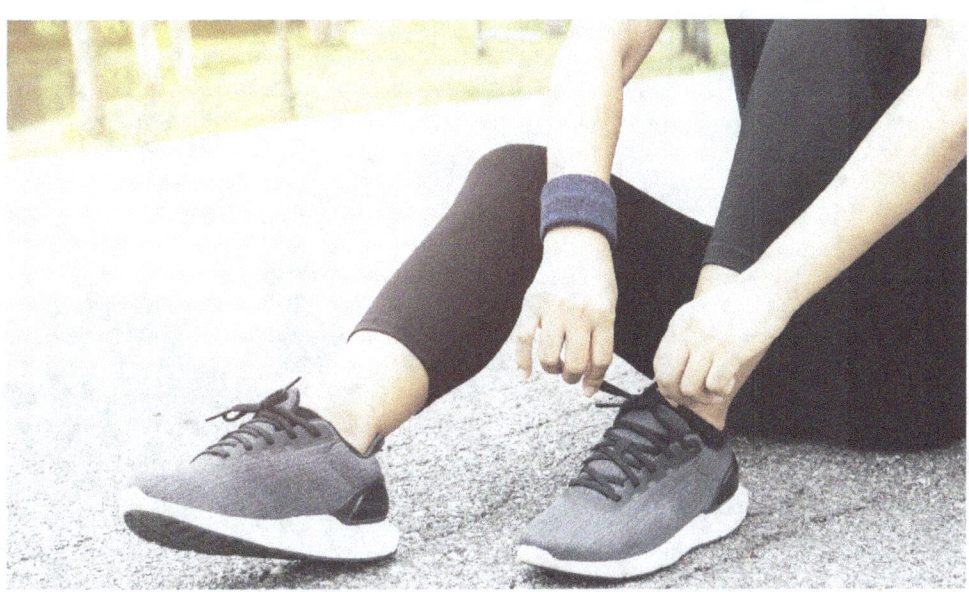

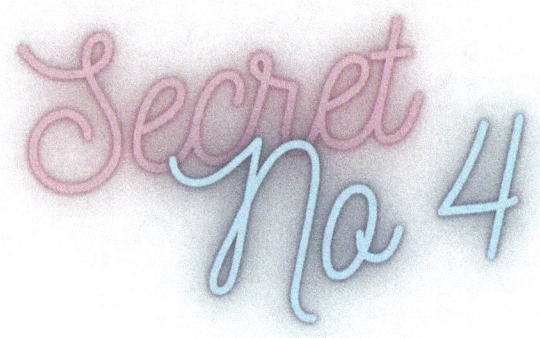

PRACTICE SLEEP PRESERVATION TECHNIQUES # SUGAR CRAVINGS ARE WORSE WHEN WE SLEEP BADLY

Our Sleep Hormone Melatonin needs to be looked after and respected to help us Sleep better and studies have shown help us to better resist cravings for Sugar and Carbs that we get when we are tired. This will help you sleep better and have less night wakings. If you go to bed before 22.30 as apposed to anytime afterwards you will have a better natural peak of this 'Sleep Hormone' to help you drift off easier and sleep better Studies have shown. Keep your screen time and snacks limited in the couple of hours before bed to encourage HGH (Human Growth Hormone) and reduce Insulin Spikes by going into your natural Night time Fasting. Poor Sleep can also be caused by Magnesuim deficiency so look to include foods that are rich in this mineral such as Seeds, Nuts (if you can eat them. And Beans.

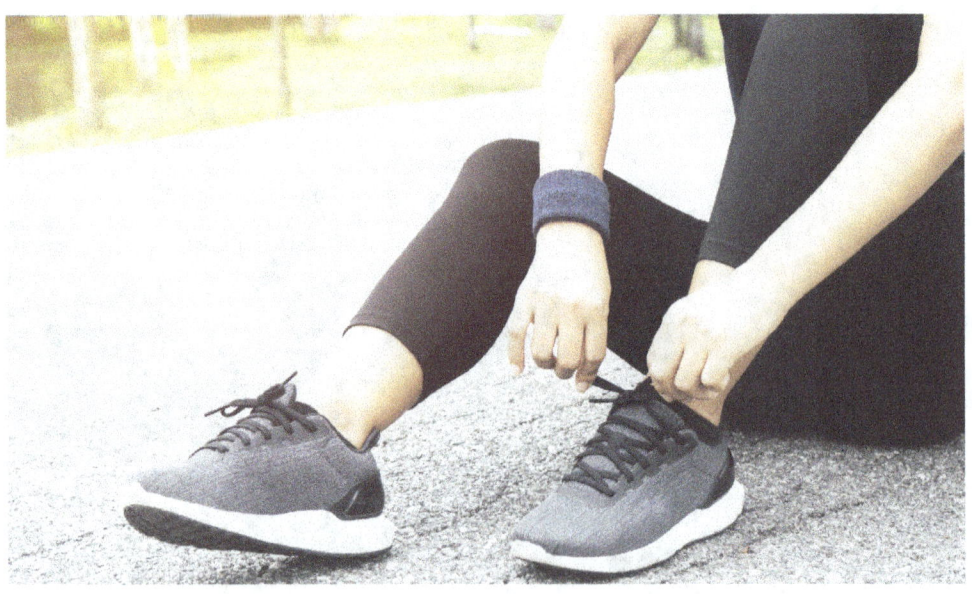

What to watch out for in your Ingredients: Corn Syrup/Fructose

Even in Low Sugar or Sugar replacement Foods be very wary of processed 'Fructose' or Corn Syrup. Research shows a link between the introduction of this Sweetner and the increase in Type 2 Diabetes . To give you some context. Diabetes was actually a rare disease back in the 1900's before we had access to processed foods and our consumption of Sugar and Sweeteners was far less.

The Studies show when Fructose was introduced in the 1960's and usage in processed foods was increased by 1000% in the 70's . During which time there was 800% increase surge in Diabetes cases.

It not just had an immediate effect on Blood Sugars strangely it can also cause spikes some time after it is consumed.

The pharmaceutical giants market for Diabetes drugs alone is a $30 billion dollar per year industry. For a disease that only came into existence when we started to consume Sugar and Sweetners.

Scientists have also warned of the 'adverse effect' of Aspartame on our Health for over 40 years- a very popular Sweetner found especially in soft drinks.

Unfortunately most Processed Food Product Producers are still putting Profits before People since it pays off for them for us to be addicted to Sugar since we will naturally buy more goods.

Even though **studies have shown than cutting just 20% of Sugar from processed foods could prevent 500,000 deaths.** We need to look after ourselves.

But is it really realistic and viable to go completely Sugar Free?

Is this helping to put you off Sugar yet?

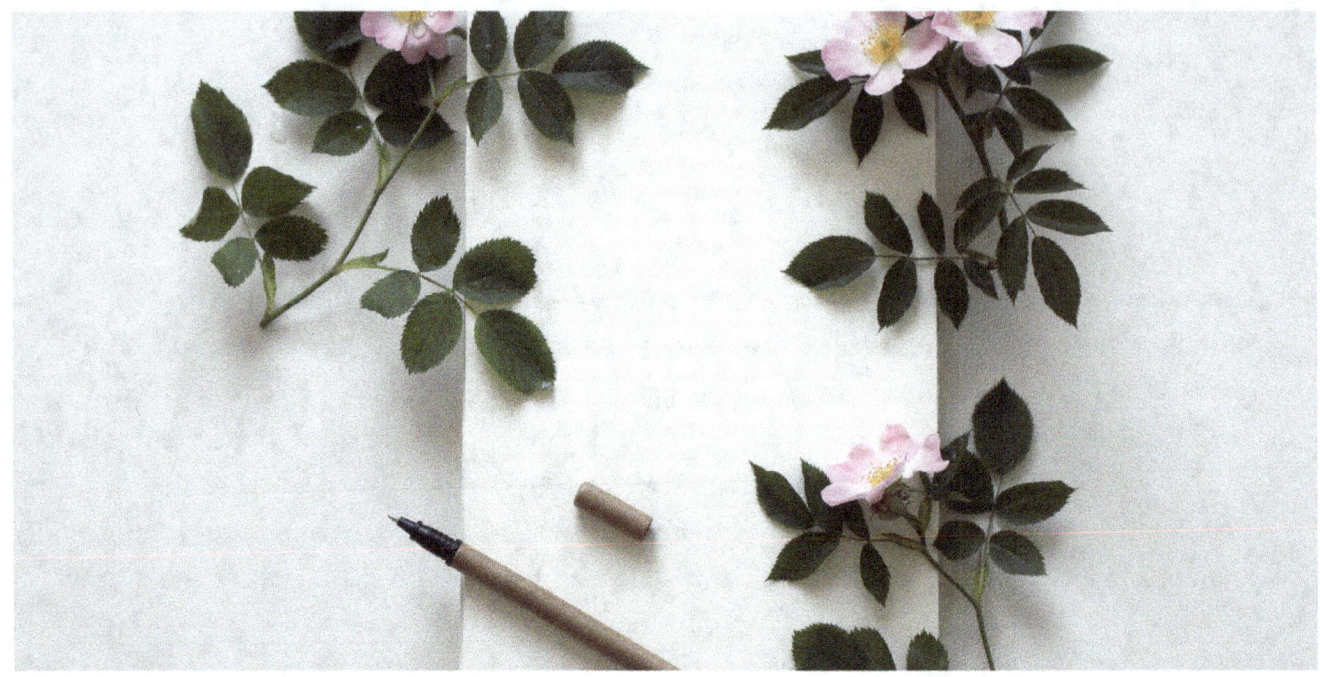

Your Own Plan of Action!..

In the next section we have a Pre Conception Plan Guide for those that are TTC skip on to this!. However if you are not TTC. At this point many women are ready to join my online Hormone Health Plan course to go deeper into each area and get help to create a more robust plan for their own journey. I have a bonus offer for you to join the 'detox' element of the plan for a special discount for completing this guide.

You can access the waiting list for the next course here by contacting me at: mymyoplan@gmail.com or go to www.HormoneHealthBliss.com

What's Next?

Congratulations on getting to the end of this guide it is now time to sit down with your note book or journal and set out how you are going to implement all of the areas in your own plan. Or you can join us on the full course and we will go through your planning and implementation together! Also join the tribe!

www.instagram.com/EmpoweredovariesTribe

Are you TTC?
Welcome to Pre-Conception Planning!

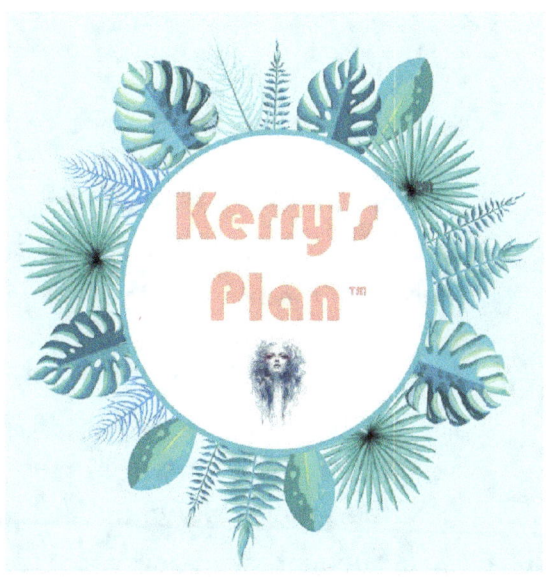

Here is a basic overview of my own pre-conception plan to optimise fertility and what steps I took to re-balance my hormones and this is also where you formulate your own plan to bring the information we already covered in this book to life, and how it can work for you personally. So get your notebook or journal out to start creating your own plan!
At this point many women are ready to join my online pre-conception plan course to go deeper into each area and get help to create a more robust plan for their own journey.
You can do this here: kerrysplan.com

Five Step
Pre-Conception Plan Strategy Framework

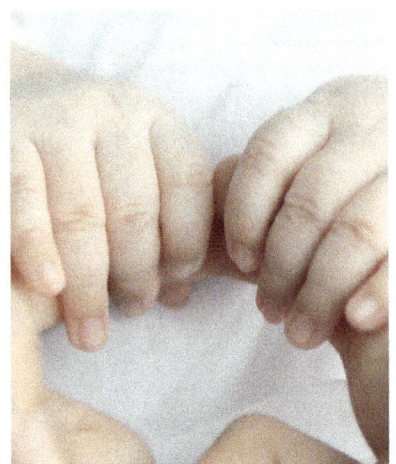

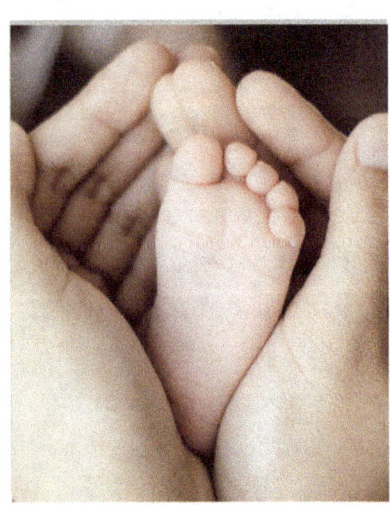

STEP 1

- Where are you currently?

- Which health checks and tests have you had so far?

- The same for your partner? Could their Health and Lifestyle be hampering Sperm quality? And are they on any medication that could affect their Sperm?

- Complete a stress test analysis - we have questionnaires to evaluate your stress levels and hormone type in the plan course. Otherwise sit down and list how you can reduce stresses and your most common moods on a daily basis.

STEP 2

- Begin fertility detox

- Balance hormones and reduce EDCs

- Clear out endocrine disruptors in your home environment as much as possible.

- Reduce sugar
- Follow the plan's melatonin maximiser sleep checklist

Five Step
Pre-Conception Plan Strategy
Framework

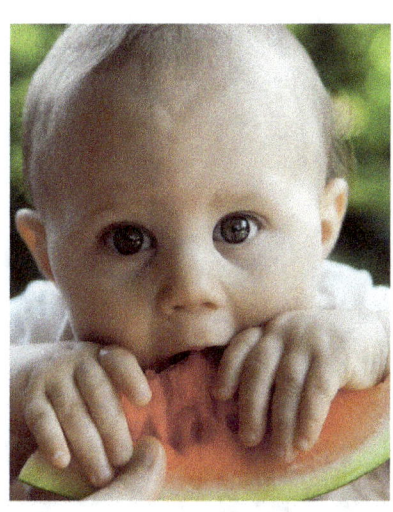

STEP 3

- Focus on nutrition and nourishment

- Start a fertility focused eating plan.

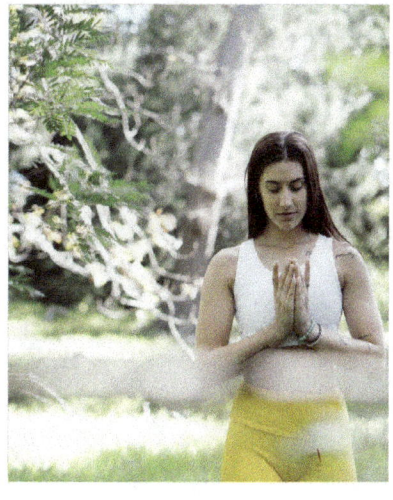

STEP 4

- Focus on supporting and working with your bodies natural energy levels.
Balance exercise by following the plan's guide to optimum levels guided throughout your cycle. Taking up fertility yoga and meditation can help relax and re-balance.

Five Step
Pre-Conception Plan Strategy
Framework

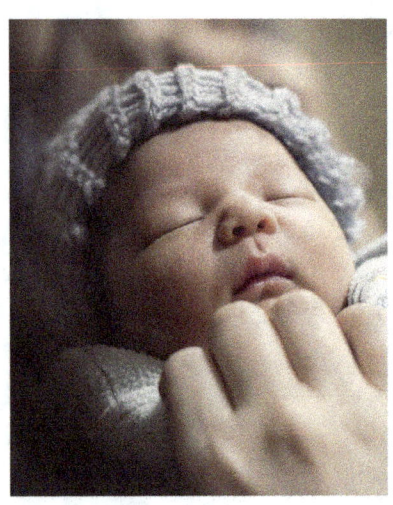

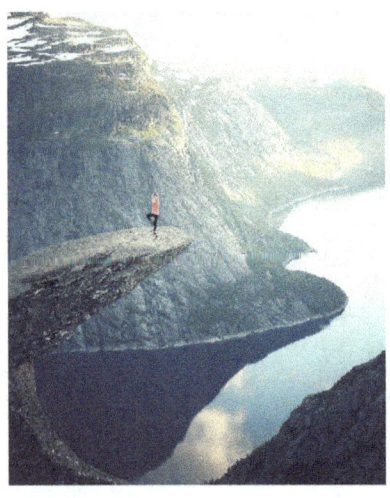

STEP 5

- Make time for mental health - mindset and stress reduction

- Revisit your stress test analysis. finding balance, changing lifestyle habits all help you to get into alignment with a more fertile mindset.

This is when women say they just start to feel really 'great'
- healthier and more in control of their bodies.
So now is the time to maximise this mindset by focusing on how far you have come and staying in this way
of living! It will benefit your long term health and hormone balance!
Healthy Hormones = Happy Lives!

At this point many women are ready to join my online pre-conception plan course to go deeper into each area and get help to create a more robust plan for their own journey.
You can do this here: kerrysplan.com